ALVEOLAR CAPILLARY DYSPLASIA DIET

Personalized Diet Strategies, Nutrient Essentials, and Flavorful Recipes Backed by Practical Tips and Expert Advice For Healing

Dr. Holmgren Alfred

The book "(ALVEOLAR CAPILLARY DYSPLASIA DIET) With Expert Guidance" is a valuable resource for anyone attempting to navigate the challenging landscape of alveolar capillary dysplasia (ACD).

This book takes the reader on a journey of understanding via painstaking detail and knowledgeable insight, offering priceless tools for both patients and caregivers.

Fundamentally, this book explores the complicated network of ACD, revealing its intricacies with accuracy and clarity.

The thorough understanding that readers gain from this detailed exploration of the condition's fundamentals, symptoms, causes, and diagnosis serves as the cornerstone for making well-informed decisions.

The narrative of the book revolves around the importance of diet in managing ACD. Acknowledging the significant influence of nutrition on health outcomes, the book clarifies the need to implement a customized dietary strategy. Readers are guided through the complex landscape of nutritional goals, issues, and the possible advantages of dietary treatments through the perspective of expertise.

Knowing is power when it comes to nutrition, and this book covers every important vitamin that is crucial for people with ACD. Every nutrient—from protein to vitamins and minerals—is carefully examined, enabling readers to make decisions that will best serve their health and well-being.

The book, however, goes beyond academic comprehension and instead uses the creation of balanced meal programs to transform information into practical actions. With an emphasis on customized methods, meal planning techniques, and useful advice for grocery shopping and meal preparation, readers are equipped to confidently take control of their dietary journey.

Furthermore, the book goes beyond nutrition to explore lifestyle factors and support networks that are essential for overall health. Readers are guided towards a path of empowerment and resilience through various means such as stress management strategies and the significance of obtaining support from healthcare professionals and support groups.

"(ALVEOLAR CAPILLARY DYSPLASIA DIET) With Expert Guidance" is more than just a book; for people struggling with ACD, it is a lifeline that provides information, hope, and support along the way to improved health and a higher standard of living.

This book, with its abundance of knowledge, helpful advice, and steadfast support, is a monument to the strength of empowerment and education in the face of hardship.

Moreover, the author makes no endorsements or recommendations regarding any person, entity, website, product, association, or other names mentioned or referenced in this work.

You consequently absolutely assume all risk associated with any reliance you may have on such material.

The use of the information included in this book may result in loss, harm, or damage for which the author is not liable.

It is recommended that readers carry out independent research and consult experts when needed.

You accept that you have read, understood, and agree to abide by this disclaimer by reading this book.

You should not use or rely on any material in this book if you disagree with any aspect of this disclaimer.

This disclaimer could change at any time, without prior warning. Please check this page from time to time for any updates or changes.

CHAPTER 1
UNDERSTANDING ALVEOLAR CAPILLARY DYSPLASIA

Overview Of ACD:

The rare and deadly developmental condition known as Alveolar Capillary Dysplasia (ACD) primarily affects the pulmonary vasculature and is characterized by defective alveolar-capillary membrane formation. Usually affecting newborns or infants, this illness causes severe respiratory distress and frequently ends in mortality in the first month of life.

The primary pathology is the deformity of the pulmonary blood vessels, specifically the alveolar capillaries, which are essential for lung gas exchange. Because of this deformity, those who are impacted have severe hypoxemia and respiratory failure, which makes treatment extremely difficult. Due to its high mortality rate and constrained therapeutic choices, ACD, despite its rarity, is a serious problem for neonatologists.

Alveolar Capillary Dysplasia's precise etiology is still unknown; most instances are thought to be sporadic and lack known genetic or environmental factors.

On the other hand, new studies have linked genetic factors—namely, mutations in the FOXF1 gene on chromosome 16q24.1—to the pathophysiology of ACD. This gene's mutations impair healthy lung development, resulting in the establishment of atypical alveolar capillaries and eventual respiratory failure. Furthermore, a few risk factors have been suggested as possible contributors to the development of ACD, including exposure to environmental contaminants or maternal smoking during pregnancy. To precisely understand the mechanics behind the onset of this uncommon condition and pinpoint the precise risk factors that may predispose people to its development, more research is necessary.

When alveolar capillary dysplasia initially manifests clinically, it usually causes severe respiratory distress in the first few hours or days of life following delivery.

Babies with ACD have symptoms such as tachypnea, cyanosis, and refractory hypoxemia, which are signs of severe lung damage related to gas exchange. Signs of pulmonary hypertension, such as right ventricular hypertrophy and high pulmonary artery pressure, frequently accompany these respiratory symptoms.

The diagnosis of ACD is based on a combination of imaging techniques, lung tissue collected through biopsy or autopsy, and histological analysis. High-resolution CT of the chest can show distinctive findings like reduced or absent pulmonary vasculature, and histological examination can show the characteristic thickened interstitial tissue and deficient pulmonary veins that are indicative of aberrant alveolar capillary development.

Options For Treatment And Difficulties:

Because Alveolar Capillary Dysplasia is uncommon and severe, managing it presents several difficulties. As of right now, ACD cannot be cured; instead, supportive care is the mainstay of therapeutic measures aimed at reducing respiratory symptoms and improving oxygenation.

To sustain appropriate oxygenation and give respiratory support to afflicted neonates, mechanical ventilation and extracorporeal membrane oxygenation (ECMO) are often utilized techniques.

The majority of infants die from respiratory failure despite intensive therapies; therefore the prognosis is still bleak. Targeted therapy development, which aims to treat the underlying vascular abnormalities in ACD, is an area of active study with potential benefits for affected patients.

Furthermore, improvements in prenatal screening and genetic testing may make it easier to identify ACD early in at-risk pregnancies, allowing for prompt interventions and individualized treatment plans. The prognosis for newborns with Alveolar Capillary Dysplasia is still uncertain despite these efforts, which emphasizes the need for more study to fully understand this debilitating condition and create cutting-edge treatment strategies that will enhance patient outcomes.

In conclusion, alveolar capillary dysplasia is an uncommon and sometimes fatal lung condition that causes aberrant alveolar-capillary membrane formation, which puts afflicted newborns at risk for severe respiratory distress. Although the precise origins of ACD are yet unknown, environmental variables and genetics may play a role in the disease's pathophysiology. Optimizing patient care and implementing appropriate therapies need early detection and diagnosis of ACD. Even though there are now few treatment options available, research efforts are continuing, so there is hope for future breakthroughs in the management of this difficult condition.

CHAPTER 2
DIET'S IMPACT ON ACD MANAGEMENT

The multidimensional approach titled

"The Role of Diet in Managing Alveolar Capillary Dysplasia (ACD)" acknowledges the importance of nutrition in providing support to patients suffering from this uncommon and intricate pulmonary vascular condition. Because of its effects on pulmonary circulation and lung function, ACD poses special problems that call for specialized dietary treatments in addition to medical care. It is essential to comprehend the role that nutrition plays in managing

ACD (2.1) to maximize patient outcomes and quality of life.

When it comes to maintaining general health and well-being, especially in people with long-term medical problems like ACD, nutrition is crucial. Beyond simple nourishment, nutrition has a critical role in managing ACD. It provides vital nutrients, supports metabolic functions, and reduces oxidative stress and inflammation.

To prevent potential consequences from ACD, adequate nutrition is necessary for immune system stimulation, growth and development promotion, and maintenance of good respiratory function.

Tailored dietary changes can also improve overall prognosis, reduce symptoms, and increase tolerance to treatment modalities.

To maintain lung health and general well-being, addressing particular dietary demands and optimizing nutrient intake are at the center of nutritional goals and concerns (2.2) in the management of ACD. Adequate energy intake is essential to sustain metabolic demands and guarantee proper growth trajectories in afflicted persons, especially babies, and children, given the possible influence of ACD on growth and development. Additionally, fulfilling metabolic demands and promoting tissue regeneration and repair depends on paying attention to the macronutrient composition, which includes protein, carbs, and fats. Sufficient intake of micronutrients, which include vitamins, minerals, and antioxidants, is also essential for enhancing immune response, lowering oxidative stress, and fostering vascular health in people with ACD.

Dietary treatments (2.3) have a range of potential benefits in the management of

ACD, encompassing both physiological and clinical outcomes. Dietary techniques that are specifically tailored to an individual's needs may be able to improve respiratory outcomes and mitigate pulmonary vascular dysfunction by modulating inflammatory pathways, reducing oxidative stress, and enhancing endothelial function.

Additionally, individualized dietary adjustments can maximize nutritional status, boost treatment tolerance, and improve overall quality of life for those with ACD. Additionally, through focused dietary alterations aimed at symptom management and disease prevention, dietary treatments may help prevent or manage comorbidities typically associated with ACD, such as pulmonary hypertension or gastroesophageal reflux disease (GERD).

In conclusion, diet plays a complex role in managing Alveolar Capillary Dysplasia (ACD). It supports general health and well-being, addresses particular nutritional goals and considerations, and maximizes the potential advantages of dietary interventions to improve patient outcomes and quality of life. Individuals with ACD can enhance their overall prognosis, reduce symptoms, and better manage their illness with customized dietary regimens, underscoring the critical role that nutrition plays in holistic ACD therapy.

CHAPTER 3
IMPORTANT NUTRIENTS FOR PATIENTS WITH ACD

Important Nutrients for Patients with Alveolar Capillary Dysplasia (ACD): These nutrients are essential for both treating the disease and maintaining general health.

For those with ACD, protein is a necessary macronutrient because it is vital to tissue growth and repair. Since the muscles around the lungs aid in breathing efficiency, maintaining muscle mass and fostering healthy lung function depend on an adequate protein intake.

Patients should concentrate on including in their diets lean meats, poultry, fish, eggs, dairy products, lentils, and tofu, as well as other high-quality protein sources.

These foods high in protein supply the essential amino acids required for many physiological functions, such as the synthesis of enzymes and the immune system. However, it's crucial to closely control protein intake because too much of it can impair kidney function in those with weakened cardiovascular and pulmonary systems.

 ACD patients' diets must include fats as well because they are a concentrated source of energy and help absorb fat-soluble vitamins. However not all fats are created equal, and patients must minimize their intake of trans and saturated fats, which can worsen cardiovascular problems and cause inflammation, and focus instead on beneficial fats. Unsaturated fats have anti-inflammatory qualities and may help reduce inflammation linked to ACD. In particular, omega-3 fatty acids are present in walnuts, flaxseeds, chia seeds, and fatty fish. Furthermore, adding monounsaturated fat sources like nuts, avocados, and olive oil can help people with ACD feel better overall and improve their hearts.

The body uses carbohydrates as its main energy source and needs them to support many physiological processes as well as optimal energy levels. ACD patients should concentrate on ingesting complex carbs since they offer a steady energy release and contain important nutrients including fiber, vitamins, and minerals. Not all carbohydrates are digested similarly, though. Excellent sources of complex carbs include whole grains, fruits, vegetables, and legumes.

For people with ACD, these foods should make up the majority of their carbohydrate consumption. In addition to giving energy, these meals support digestive health and satiety, two important factors for individuals managing ACD and related symptoms.

Minerals and vitamins are vital parts of the diet for ACD sufferers because they support immunological function and general health. For those with ACD, maintaining optimal health and supporting numerous physiological processes requires an adequate intake of minerals like calcium, magnesium, potassium, and zinc, as well as vitamins like A, C, D, E, and K. To address certain deficits or maximize nutrient status, patients may require individualized supplementation or dietary adjustments because their needs may differ.

For people with ACD, the best way to guarantee appropriate vitamin and mineral intake is through a diverse and balanced diet that includes a wide variety of nutrient-dense foods. Healthcare specialists should guide supplementation based on the needs of each patient and their medical history.

For people with ACD, fluids and hydration are crucial factors to take into account because proper hydration is necessary to sustain cardiovascular health, maintain lung function at its best, and enhance general well-being. Hydration is vital for patients to maintain throughout the day, as dehydration can worsen symptoms including weariness and dyspnea. While fresh juices, herbal teas, and broths can also help increase overall fluid consumption, water is still the greatest option for hydration. However, as they might exacerbate symptoms and contribute to dehydration, patients with ACD should llmit or avoid excessive use of caffeinated and sugary drinks. Pale yellow pee indicates sufficient hydration, thus keeping an eye on the color and output of your urine can assist in determining your level of hydration. Additionally, to find out specific recommendations for fluid intake based on individual needs and medical considerations, people with ACD should speak with their healthcare professional.

vital foods such as protein, lipids, carbs, vitamins, minerals, and liquids are critical for maintaining general health and controlling symptoms in people with alveolar capillary dysplasia. For ACD patients to achieve their nutrient needs and maintain optimal well-being, a diversified, balanced diet rich in nutrient-dense foods is essential. Individualized dietary plans that are supervised by medical specialists and customized to meet specific needs can help maximize nutritional intake and assist in managing symptoms in ACD sufferers.

CHAPTER 4
CREATING A BALANCED ACD DIET PLAN

Tailored Nutrition Programs:

The rare and serious pulmonary condition known as Alveolar Capillary Dysplasia (ACD) is typified by aberrant capillary growth surrounding the alveoli in the lungs. Because of this, people with ACD frequently need specific dietary therapies to effectively manage their illness. It's critical to take into account each patient's particular nutritional requirements and obstacles while creating a balanced ACD diet plan. This calls for the development of customized diet regimens that take into account unique food choices, lifestyle considerations, and health issues.

 For those with ACD, individualized diet programs usually entail a thorough evaluation of their present health status, taking into account variables including age, weight, medical history, and any coexisting conditions. Personalized dietary advice can be informed by the evaluation of a patient's metabolic irregularities or nutritional inadequacies by licensed dietitians or nutritionists, among other healthcare professionals, through the use of specialized tests. Healthcare professionals can develop customized diet regimens that maximize nutrient intake while reducing potential dietary triggers or exacerbating variables for symptoms of ACD by accounting for these unique features.

Additionally, nutrient-dense foods that support respiratory health, such as fruits, vegetables, whole grains, lean proteins, and healthy fats, should be given priority in customized diet regimens for individuals with ACD. Essential vitamins, minerals, antioxidants, and phytonutrients included in these foods support immune system function, lung function, and general health. Dietary recommendations may include containing particular nutrients, such as omega-3 fatty acids, vitamin D, vitamin C, and magnesium, which are proven to be important for lung health. People with ACD may be able to enhance lung development, oxygenation, and tissue regeneration by including these nutrient-dense foods in their diet, which may slow the disease's progression and enhance quality of life.

Strategies For Meal Planning:

To ensure that people with ACD satisfy their nutritional needs, follow dietary recommendations, and manage potential dietary triggers, meal planning is an essential part of a balanced diet plan. Careful consideration of nutrient composition, portion sizes, meal timing, and food preparation techniques are essential components of effective meal-planning strategies for ACD. Individuals can improve overall health outcomes, limit symptom exacerbation, and optimize their nutritional consumption by implementing these techniques.

Setting nutrient-dense meals as a top priority in meal planning for people with ACD is important because they include vital vitamins, minerals, and antioxidants that support the immune system and respiratory health. This entails arranging meals and snacks throughout the day to incorporate a range of fruits, vegetables, whole grains, lean proteins, and healthy fats. People can make sure they get enough of the essential nutrients by emphasizing nutrient-rich meals and reducing their intake of processed foods, added sugars, and bad fats, which can worsen the symptoms of ACD or cause other health problems.

Portion control and meal frequency are crucial factors to take into account when organizing meals for people with ACD. People may benefit from eating smaller, more frequent meals and snacks rather than large, heavier ones since dietary factors may have an impact on symptoms of ACD. This strategy can help control symptoms including exhaustion, lack of appetite, and shortness of breath by preventing overeating, easing gastrointestinal distress, and stabilizing blood sugar levels. Furthermore, portion management can assist people in avoiding overindulging in calories and maintaining a healthy weight, both of which are critical for treating complications associated with ACD, such as respiratory failure and pulmonary hypertension.

Controlling Portion Size and Meal Frequency:

When creating a balanced ACD diet plan, portion control, and meal frequency are crucial factors to take into account because they have a big impact on how well symptoms are managed, how much nourishment is consumed, and the general state of health.

Smaller, more frequent meals and snacks may help reduce gastrointestinal distress, balance blood sugar, and promote normal respiratory function in people with ACD.

Through mindful eating practices and portion control, people can enhance their nutritional intake, efficiently manage symptoms, and live better.

Portion management is regulating how much food is eaten at each meal and snack to make sure it satisfies dietary recommendations and each person's unique nutritional requirements. To determine the proper serving sizes, this may entail measuring portion sizes using instruments like measuring cups, food scales, or visual cues. To reduce overeating and encourage better digestion, people can also employ techniques like sharing entrees at restaurants, cutting meals into smaller pieces, and staying away from big servings. People can prevent obesity, pulmonary hypertension, and respiratory failure, maintain a healthy weight, and lower their chance of developing complications connected to ACD by adopting portion management.

Meal frequency is essential for controlling ACD symptoms and maximizing dietary intake, in addition to quantity control. People may profit more from eating smaller, more frequent meals and snacks throughout the day as opposed to large, heavy meals that are consumed infrequently.

This strategy helps lessen gastrointestinal distress, avoid overtaxing the digestive system, and supply a consistent energy source for bodily functions like breathing and exercise. People can control blood sugar levels, sustain energy levels, and avoid ACD symptoms like weakness, exhaustion, and dizziness by distributing meals and snacks equally throughout the day.

Getting Used to Dietary Restrictions and Preferences:

Creating a balanced, pleasurable, and individually tailored ACD diet plan requires careful consideration of food preferences and limits. Although there may be dietary guidelines for ACD sufferers to promote respiratory health and manage symptoms, it's important to understand that meal planning and food choices can also be influenced by cultural customs, dietary preferences, and food allergies or intolerances. Through recognition of these variables and cooperation with medical professionals, people can create adaptable eating plans that satisfy their particular dietary needs and constraints while maintaining a focus on symptom relief and adequate nutrition.

Concentrating on nutrient-dense foods that fit with unique dietary patterns and cultural preferences is one way to adjust to dietary preferences and limits in ACD management. To meet their protein demands, people who follow vegetarian or vegan diets, for instance, might focus on plant-based protein sources such as beans, lentils, tofu, and nuts. They can also incorporate a range of fruits, vegetables, whole grains, and healthy fats to create a balanced diet.

In a similar vein, people with food allergies or intolerances can find appropriate replacements and alternatives to stay away from trigger foods while still getting the nourishment they need.

Working with a trained dietitian or nutritionist, who may offer individualized advice and assistance to successfully negotiate dietary preferences and constraints, may also be beneficial for those with ACD.

These medical specialists can assist people in making appropriate food choices, organizing well-balanced meals, and addressing any issues or difficulties with diet control. People can create a personalized ACD diet plan that supports their particular dietary needs and preferences and promotes maximum health and well-being by working with an experienced healthcare team.

creating a balanced ACD diet plan necessitates a customized strategy that considers dietary choices or constraints, meal planning techniques, portion control, and individual nutritional needs. People with ACD can maximize their nutritional intake, effectively manage symptoms, and enhance their overall quality of life by emphasizing nutrient-dense meals, exercising portion control, and adjusting to their dietary patterns. Working together with medical professionals, such as nutritionists or registered dietitians, can improve dietary management even further and help ACD sufferers achieve long-term health benefits.

CHAPTER 5
FOODS TO ADD TO AN ACD DIET

Lean Protein Sources: Essential for the immune system and tissue repair as well as general health maintenance, protein supports several body processes.

Lean protein sources are especially crucial in the context of an Alveolar Capillary

Dysplasia (ACD) diet because of their decreased fat content, which lessens the strain on the cardiovascular system.

Lean pig or beef cuts, seafood, tofu, skinless chicken, and lentils are a few examples of lean protein sources.

These protein sources offer the vital amino acids required for the body's processes of growth and repair without contributing excessive amounts of cholesterol or saturated fat, which might worsen the cardiovascular problems linked to ACD.

A varied food intake is ensured by including a range of lean protein sources, all while reducing the risk of adverse effects on cardiovascular health.

Healthy Fats and Oils: Although fats are sometimes vilified in diet talks, some kinds of fats are crucial for preserving good health, particularly when it comes to treating an illness like ACD.

Because they lower inflammation and raise cholesterol, healthy fats like monounsaturated and polyunsaturated fats are essential for maintaining cardiovascular health. Avocados, nuts, seeds, olive oil, avocados, and fatty fish like mackerel and salmon are good sources of healthful fats and oils. Essential elements found in these fats include omega-3 and omega-6 fatty acids, which have been linked to several health advantages, such as enhanced vascular function and a lower risk of cardiovascular illnesses. But moderation is essential since even good fats have a high calorie density and consuming too much of them can cause weight gain, which puts stress on the cardiovascular system.

Whole Grains and High-Fibre Foods: Because they can help to maintain cardiovascular health and control blood sugar levels, whole grains, and high-fiber foods are essential parts of an ACD diet. While processed grains are depleted of their bran and germ layers, whole grains maintain their fiber content and offer vital elements such as antioxidants, vitamins, and minerals. Furthermore, dietary fiber is essential for maintaining digestive health and avoiding constipation, which is a typical issue for people with ACD.

Oats, brown rice, quinoa, whole wheat bread, and barley are a few types of whole grains. A consistent supply of nutrients is ensured by including a range of whole grains and foods high in fiber. This also encourages satiety, which can help with weight control and cardiovascular health in general.

Fruits and Vegetables: An ACD diet must include fruits and vegetables since they are excellent providers of vitamins, minerals, antioxidants, and dietary fiber.

These nutrient-dense meals support proper vascular function, lower inflammation, and raise blood pressure in addition to providing vital nutrients for general health and cardiovascular health. A varied nutritional intake can be achieved by including a range of colorful fruits and vegetables since different colors denote the presence of different phytonutrients with distinct health advantages.

Berries, leafy greens, citrus fruits, tomatoes, carrots, and bell peppers are a few examples of healthy fruits and vegetables. Eating a variety of fruits and vegetables in their fresh, frozen, or canned states (without added sugars or syrups) guarantees a sufficient intake of nutrients while enhancing the taste and texture of food.

 Dairy and Dairy Alternatives: Calcium, vitamin D, and protein are vital nutrients that are critical for healthy bones and general well-being. Dairy products and their substitutes can be excellent sources of these nutrients. Dairy products should be used with caution by those with ACD, though, as some of them—especially those heavy in saturated fats—may make cardiovascular problems worse.

In these situations, choosing low-fat or fat-free dairy products and looking into plant-based milk substitutes such as fortified almond or soy milk can be helpful.

These substitutes offer vital nutrients without the possible harm to cardiovascular health that comes from consuming large amounts of saturated fat. Incorporating fermented dairy products, such as kefir and yogurt, can also supply probiotics, which boost immunity and gut health.

Herbs, spices, and flavor enhancers: In restricted diets such as ACD, herbs, spices, and flavor enhancers are essential for improving the flavor and palatability of food. Herbs and spices provide a variety of flavors without adding too much sodium, although salt and sodium should be avoided because of their possible effects on blood pressure and cardiovascular health. Furthermore, a wide variety of herbs and spices include anti-inflammatory and antioxidant qualities that can help cardiovascular health by lowering inflammation and oxidative stress. Herbs and spices that are tasty include cumin, cinnamon, ginger, turmeric, basil, and rosemary. ACD dieters can prioritize cardiovascular health and overall well-being while preparing delicious and gratifying meals by experimenting with different herbs, spices, and flavor enhancers.

CHAPTER 6
FOODS TO LIMIT OR AVOID

Foods High In Sodium:

Foods classified as high-sodium belong to a group of dietary items that have higher concentrations of sodium chloride, or salt. Restricting sodium intake is especially important while addressing Alveolar Capillary Dysplasia (ACD), a rare congenital condition that affects how lung blood vessels form. Because sodium causes fluid retention and raises blood pressure, consuming too much of it might worsen ACD symptoms including respiratory distress. Processed meats, canned soups, fast food, salty snacks, and some sauces are examples of foods high in sodium. Within an ACD-specific diet plan, these foods should be consumed in moderation or not at all.

Rather, the focus should be on choosing healthy, fresh meals and adding taste with spices, herbs, and other low-sodium substitutes. This dietary strategy lowers the risk of hypertension and its associated problems, which not only improves general cardiovascular health but also helps manage the symptoms of ACD.

Refined And Processed Foods:

Foods that have been significantly altered from their natural state through various production procedures are referred to as processed or refined foods. These meals are often lacking in fiber and important nutrients and heavy in added sugars, bad fats, salt, and other additives. When it comes to managing ACD, these foods provide several difficulties. First of all, they aggravate ACD symptoms and impair lung function by causing inflammation and oxidative stress. Second, because of their high glycemic index, there may be variations in blood sugar levels, which could have a detrimental effect on general health and exacerbate metabolic problems. Consequently, processed and refined foods such as sugary cereals, white bread, pastries, packaged snacks, and sugary beverages should be avoided or consumed in moderation by those with ACD.

To support normal lung function and general well-being, the emphasis should instead be on complete, unprocessed foods including fruits, vegetables, whole grains, lean proteins, and healthy fats.

Sugar-Filled Foods And Drinks:

Sugary foods and drinks include a broad variety of items that either naturally contain high levels of sugar, such as fructose, glucose, and sucrose, or have added sugars. Candy, pastries, drinks with added sugar, sweets, and a lot of processed foods are among them. Sugary foods and drinks should be consumed in moderation when managing ACD because of their negative impact on inflammation and metabolic health.

Consuming large amounts of sugar has been associated with insulin resistance, obesity, cardiovascular disease, and other metabolic problems. These conditions can worsen the symptoms of Acute Onset Disorder and affect lung function.

 Additionally, sugary foods frequently lack fiber and other vital elements, thus impairing nutritional status. As a result, people with ACD should emphasize complete, nutrient-dense foods and choose naturally sweet foods like fresh fruit, unsweetened yogurt, and, if necessary, tiny amounts of honey or maple syrup.

Reduced sugar intake and an emphasis on whole-food, balanced options can help people with ACD better manage their illness and promote general health.

Possible Intolerances Or Allergens:

Foods that, in certain people, may cause allergic reactions or unfavorable digestive symptoms are referred to as potential allergens or intolerances. Nuts, shellfish, dairy, eggs, soy, and gluten-containing cereals are among the common allergies. Identifying and avoiding any allergies or intolerances is crucial for managing ACD because it prevents needless inflammation and pain, which can worsen symptoms and jeopardize general health. Furthermore, underlying food sensitivities or intolerances in certain ACD sufferers may worsen inflammation or cause gastrointestinal problems. As such, individualized nutrition therapy is critical, entailing a thorough evaluation of each person's unique food triggers and, if required, the application of an elimination diet. People with ACD can maximize their nutritional intake, boost immunological function, and reduce symptom exacerbation by avoiding known allergies or intolerances and focusing on natural, minimally processed meals. Additionally, seeking advice and support from a registered dietitian or other healthcare professional who specializes in food allergies and intolerances can be very helpful in helping people with ACD navigate dietary restrictions and maximize their nutritional intake.

CHAPTER 7
RECIPES AND IDEAS FOR MEALS

Meal Ideas and Recipes: The details of creating a customized diet plan for people with alveolar capillary dysplasia (ACD) are covered in this section of "Alveolar Capillary Dysplasia Diet". Acknowledging the critical role that nutrition plays in the management of this illness, this chapter provides in-depth information on meal planning, recipe development, and cooking methods that are suited to the unique dietary requirements of individuals with ACD. This section tries to equip patients and caregivers with useful ways to achieve optimal health and well-being by highlighting the significance of a balanced diet rich in necessary nutrients while meeting individual tastes and limits.

Breakfast alternatives: When it comes to breakfast alternatives, the goal is to offer healthy, stimulating meal options that meet the nutritional needs of people with ACD. This section emphasizes the value of a healthy breakfast and provides a wide variety of breakfast options, from protein-rich smoothies with vitamins and minerals to hearty oatmeal bowls loaded with fiber and antioxidants. ACD patients can enhance overall health and vitality by boosting their metabolism and maintaining energy levels throughout the day by including nutritious grains, lean meats, and fresh fruits in their morning meals.

Lunch and Dinner Ideas: The chapter covers a wide range of gastronomic options for lunch and dinner that are intended to please palates and meet dietary requirements. The focus is on preparing balanced and filling meals that support optimal health and promote satiety, from colorful salads full of lean proteins and colorful veggies to hearty grain bowls stuffed with fiber and vital nutrients.

ACD patients can enjoy tasty and nutritious meals that support their overall health and illness management by consuming a range of nutrient-dense foods while eliminating processed foods and bad fats.

Snack Recommendations: Snacking is essential for sustaining energy levels and avoiding hunger-related cravings all day long. This section focuses on offering nutrient-dense, easily portable snack options to patients with ACD that complement their dietary preferences and goals. The focus is on selecting snacks that are high in protein, fiber, and healthy fats and low in artificial additives and refined sugars.

Examples of these snacks include crunchy veggie sticks with hummus, protein-packed yogurt parfaits, and homemade energy bars. ACD sufferers can easily control their hunger and cravings while providing their bodies with the necessary nutrition by making a plan ahead of time and keeping a selection of healthy snacks convenient.

example Recipes and Cooking Ideas: This section provides a variety of example recipes along with helpful cooking techniques and ideas to help ACD patients and their caretakers prepare meals.

Every recipe, which ranges from easy yet tasty soups and stews to filling meals and side dishes, is carefully designed to satisfy dietary requirements and preferences while offering a balance of macronutrients and micronutrients. Helpful cooking advice is also offered to speed up the cooking process and improve the nutritional value of meals, including portion control methods, ingredient replacements, and meal planning ideas. Cooking creativity combined with evidence-based dietary guidelines allows ACD patients to enjoy tasty, nutritious meals that help them on their path to better health and well-being.

CHAPTER 8
PRACTICAL ADVICE FOR GROCERY SHOPPING AND MEAL PLANNING

Organizing meals and navigating grocery store aisles can be important parts of meeting dietary needs, especially for people with diseases like Alveolar Capillary Dysplasia (ACD). This section offers in-depth information on successful grocery shopping and meal preparation techniques designed to specifically address the needs of people with ACD.

Reading Food Labels: For people with ACD to make educated dietary decisions, they must be able to decipher food labels. This entails closely examining labels to find important nutritional details about ingredients, serving sizes, and nutrient content.

For example, it's critical to recognize any allergies or chemicals that could aggravate symptoms. Furthermore, people might need to monitor their micronutrient levels carefully, especially those that support lung health and general well-being.

Making healthier decisions while grocery shopping can be facilitated by practical advice on how to read labels and distinguish between dangerous components and those that are healthy.

Budget-Friendly Buying Techniques: Many people and families find it difficult to balance the dietary restrictions related to ACD with a strict budget. This section provides helpful tips on how to shop for wholesome foods without going over budget. Cost-effective basics like nutritious grains, legumes, and seasonal produce should be prioritized. Other strategies include using coupons, purchasing in bulk, and taking advantage of promotions and discounts. Furthermore, advice on meal planning and using inexpensive, healthy ingredients in recipes can help people maximize their grocery budget without sacrificing the quality of their food.

Meal Preparation and Batch Cooking: These techniques can be quite helpful for people with ACD since they help them prepare meals more quickly and guarantee that they have access to healthy, home-cooked meals all week long. This section explores useful strategies and tactics for effective meal preparation, such as creating menus ahead of time, cooking large amounts of meals or components at once, and portioning and storing food appropriately for later use. People can prioritize their nutritional needs and health objectives while reducing stress and saving time by setting up a specific period each week for meal prep.

 Managing Eating Out and Social Events: Eating out or going to social events might make it harder to keep a balanced diet and follow the dietary limitations related to ACD. This section of the guide provides advice on how to handle these circumstances and still enjoy social gatherings and a variety of cuisines.

 Some advice could be to go through menus ahead of time, let servers or hosts know about any dietary restrictions, and, if possible, select customizable or allergy-friendly options. Advice on portion management and mindful eating techniques can also enable people to choose healthier options when dining out or attending social gatherings without feeling guilty or alone.

helpful hints for meal planning and grocery shopping are essential for helping people with ACD manage their nutritional needs and enhance their general health and well-being.

Through the provision of information and abilities to facilitate decision-making, manage finances, expedite meal preparation, and navigate social settings, this all-inclusive manual enables people to prioritize their dietary requirements and flourish despite the obstacles presented by their illness.

CHAPTER 9
SUPPORT AND LIFESTYLE CONSIDERATIONS

Since physical activity enhances general health and well-being, it is essential for managing Alveolar Capillary Dysplasia (ACD). Regular exercise helps to strengthen muscles, improve lung function, and improve cardiovascular health—all of which are critical for people with ACD. Walking, swimming, or cycling are examples of aerobic workouts that can help increase lung capacity and efficiency, making it easier for people to manage the respiratory difficulties brought on by ACD. Additionally, exercise helps lower the risk of obesity-related problems, maintain a healthy weight, and improve circulation—all of which are crucial for people with ACD who may develop pulmonary hypertension.

However, it's important for people with ACD to exercise carefully and under the supervision of medical specialists because intense exercise or overexertion can aggravate respiratory symptoms or cause problems.

To guarantee safe and efficient physical activity, customized exercise regimens based on each person's condition, degree of fitness, and medical background should be created in conjunction with healthcare professionals.

Techniques For Stress Management:

For those who have Alveolar Capillary Dysplasia (ACD), stress management is essential because stress can worsen symptoms and have a detrimental effect on general well-being. Stress can cause physiological reactions like elevated heart rate and shallow breathing, which can make respiratory problems worse for those with ACD.

Consequently, enhancing the quality of life and lessening the intensity of symptoms requires the adoption of efficient stress management strategies. Methods including progressive muscle relaxation, yoga, meditation, deep breathing exercises, and meditation can assist people with ACD reduce stress, becoming more relaxed, and enhancing their coping skills.

Furthermore, integrating mindfulness exercises into regular activities can support people in maintaining present-moment awareness and lowering worry related to their health. For those with ACD, it's critical to recognize stressors and create individualized plans for efficiently handling them. Joining support groups or obtaining assistance from mental health specialists can also offer helpful tools and motivation for putting stress management strategies into practice.

Looking for Assistance from Medical Professionals and Support Organizations:

For those with Alveolar Capillary Dysplasia (ACD) and their families, getting help from medical professionals and support organizations is crucial.

Throughout managing ACD, medical specialists such as pulmonologists, cardiologists, genetic counselors, and dietitians are vital in providing medical care, direction, and support. They can organize thorough care plans catered to the needs of the patient and provide insightful information about the illness, relevant resources, and treatment alternatives. Support groups also give people with ACD and their families a way to meet people who have gone through similar things, exchange knowledge, give emotional support, and get connected to local resources.

A sense of empowerment and belonging can be fostered by discussing experiences, difficulties, and triumphs with people who are aware of the intricacies of living with ACD. Additionally, support groups may plan advocacy campaigns, educational events, and fundraising activities to increase public knowledge of ACD and support studies that attempt to enhance diagnostic and treatment outcomes.

To improve their general well-being and resilience, people with ACD and their families are therefore urged to actively seek out and engage in healthcare services and support groups.

Alveolar Capillary Dysplasia (ACD) management demands careful planning, adaptation, and support from family, friends, and medical experts to balance with daily life. There are several obstacles to overcome when dealing with a chronic and complicated medical condition such as ACD. These include controlling symptoms, following treatment plans, going to doctor's appointments, and handling practical and emotional worries. As a result, people with ACD and their families must create plans for incorporating ACD management into their everyday activities without sacrificing their feeling of normalcy or quality of life.

To support general health and well-being, this may entail giving self-care practices—

such as healthy eating, enough sleep, and stress management—priority.

Furthermore, proactive participation in treatment decision-making and efficient communication with healthcare practitioners can empower people to feel in control of their condition. Navigating the difficulties of living with ACD while achieving personal and professional objectives requires flexibility, resilience, and a strong support system of family, friends, and medical experts. Notwithstanding the difficulties caused by their illness, people with ACD can endeavor to lead healthy and meaningful lives by emphasizing self-care, getting help when necessary, and taking proactive measures to manage their disease.

CHAPTER 10
ACD DIET PLAN MONITORING AND ADJUSTMENT

Frequent Evaluation Of Nutritious Status

Regular nutritional status monitoring is crucial in the context of the Alveolar Capillary Dysplasia (ACD) diet to guarantee the best possible health outcomes for those afflicted with this uncommon and possibly fatal disorder. Key nutritional factors such as macronutrient intake (carbs, proteins, and fats), micronutrient levels (vitamins and minerals), hydration state, and total caloric consumption are all systematically assessed as part of the monitoring process. Healthcare specialists, such as registered dietitians or nutritionists, who specialize in managing medical nutrition therapy for people with complicated medical disorders lIke ACD, frequently start this process with a thorough nutritional assessment.

Frequent monitoring enables the early identification of any nutritional imbalances or deficits that may result from the special dietary needs related to ACD. It also offers insightful information on how well the suggested food plan works and aids in directing changes to maximize nutritional support and advance general well-being.

Adapting Depending On Each Person's Reaction And Needs:

The ACD diet plan's efficacy depends on its capacity to adjust to the unique requirements and reactions of every patient. No two people with ACD are precisely the same, and dietary tolerances and nutritional needs can vary according to age, gender, metabolic rate, disease severity, and coexisting medical problems.

As a result, it is crucial to implement a customized strategy for diet management that considers these individual variations.

It is important to constantly monitor the patient's nutritional status, symptoms, and general health outcomes throughout time to make necessary alterations to the diet plan based on their reaction. Modifications could be required, for instance, if a patient finds it difficult to tolerate a particular cuisine or develops nutritional deficits even when following the recommended diet.

To better suit the patient's needs, this may entail changing the macronutrient composition, modifying portion sizes, adding extra nutrition support, or looking at alternate dietary options. To optimize nutritional management and enhance clinical results, regular communication between the patient, their caregivers, and healthcare practitioners is essential for spotting any problems and working together to develop creative solutions.

Interacting With Healthcare Professionals:

The effective execution of the ACD diet plan and continued management of the illness depend on good communication between patients, caregivers, and healthcare professionals. Healthcare professionals are essential in helping patients and their families navigate the dietary management process by offering evidence-based advice and continuously tracking their progress. Frequent contact enables the sharing of important details about the patient's nutritional condition, dietary preferences, compliance with the recommended diet plan, and any obstacles or issues that could come up. This makes it possible for medical professionals to provide prompt assistance, handle any problems that can prevent dietary adherence or nutritional sufficiency, and decide intelligently when to modify the diet plan. Furthermore, teamwork and trust are fostered by open and transparent communication, enabling all parties engaged in the patient's care to work together to achieve shared objectives and maximize results.

Healthcare professionals can better understand each patient's particular needs and preferences, customize dietary advice, and offer comprehensive assistance to enhance the overall health and well-being of people with ACD by keeping lines of communication open.

CONCLUSION

the Alveolar Capillary Dysplasia (ACD) diet is an essential part of the all-encompassing care plan for people with this uncommon and intricate illness.

The goal of the ACD diet is to maximize nutritional support, reduce symptoms, and enhance the overall quality of life for patients and their families through individualized diet methods, nutrient necessities, and tasty meals supported by helpful hints and professional assistance.

Successful dietary management in ACD is mostly dependent on three key ideas: continuous monitoring of nutritional status, making adjustments depending on individual response and needs, and efficient communication with healthcare specialists.

Patients can improve their nutritional outcomes, reduce complications, and strengthen their capacity to manage the difficulties brought on by this uncommon illness by following these guidelines.

To enhance long-term results for people with ACD, broaden access to specialist nutritional support, and further refine dietary guidelines, more research, collaboration, and advocacy initiatives are required.